SPOTLIGHT ON GLOBAL ISSUES

PHYSICAL HEALTH FOR ALL

Rachael Morlock

ROSEN PUBLISHING
NEW YORK

Published in 2022 by The Rosen Publishing Group, Inc.
29 East 21st Street, New York, NY 10010

First Edition

Editor: Theresa Emminizer
Book Design: Michael Flynn

Photo Credits: Cover goffkein.pro/Shutterstock.com; (series globe background) photastic/Shutterstock.com; p. 4 FatCamera/E+/Getty Images; p. 5 Jose Luis Pelaez Inc/DigitalVision/Getty Images; p. 7 DEA/A.DAGLI ORTI/De Agostini/Getty Images; p. 8 Fine Art/Corbis Historical/Getty Images; p. 9 Print Collector/Hulton Archive/Getty Images; p. 11 Popperfoto/Getty Images; p. 12 Maxx-Studio/Shutterstock.com; p. 13 Mohammed Hammoud/Getty Images; pp. 14, 15 Adam Jan Figel/Shutterstock.com; p. 16 Digital Images Studio/Shutterstock.com; p. 17 MLADEN ANTONOV/AFP/Getty Images; p. 19 (cancer cell) jovan vitanovski/Shutterstock.com; p. 19 (Rishab Jain) https://en.wikipedia.org/wiki/Rishab_Jain#/media/File:RishabJain_2018.jpg; p. 20 Hung Chung Chih/Shutterstock.com; p. 21 STR/Stringer/AFP/Getty Images; p. 22 Anna Om/Shutterstock.com; p. 23 ISSOUF SANOGO/AFP/Getty Images; p. 25 hadynyah/E+/Getty Images; p. 26 Valeri Potapova/Shutterstock.com; p. 27 OLYMPIA DE MAISMONT/AFP/Getty Images; p. 28 Andrey_Popov/Shutterstock.com; p. 29 RUTH MCDOWALL/AFP/Getty Images.

Library of Congress Cataloging-in-Publication Data

Names: Morlock, Rachael, author.
Title: Physical health for all / Rachael Morlock.
Description: New York : Rosen Publishing, [2022] | Series: Spotlight on global issues | Includes index.
Identifiers: LCCN 2020003760 | ISBN 9781725323490 (paperback) | ISBN 9781725323520 (library binding) | ISBN 9781725323506 (6 pack)
Subjects: LCSH: Health--Juvenile literature. | Hygiene--Juvenile literature.
Classification: LCC RA777 .M677 2022 | DDC 613--dc23
LC record available at https://lccn.loc.gov/2020003760

Manufactured in the United States of America

CPSIA Compliance Information: Batch #CSR22. For further information contact Rosen Publishing, New York, New York at 1-800-237-9932.

CONTENTS

CHAPTER ONE

HEALTHY GOALS

One of the most powerful ways to build a strong and thriving community is to support the physical health of its members. In the global community, many physical health challenges prevent people from living well. But new directions and discoveries in science and technology can help people live healthier lives and contribute to the best possible world.

Over 95 percent of the world's population suffers from at least one health problem. Some problems can be easily cured, while others last a long time and can lead to disability or death. Everyone should be able to access medical care when they need it, and providing accessible and effective care is a global challenge.

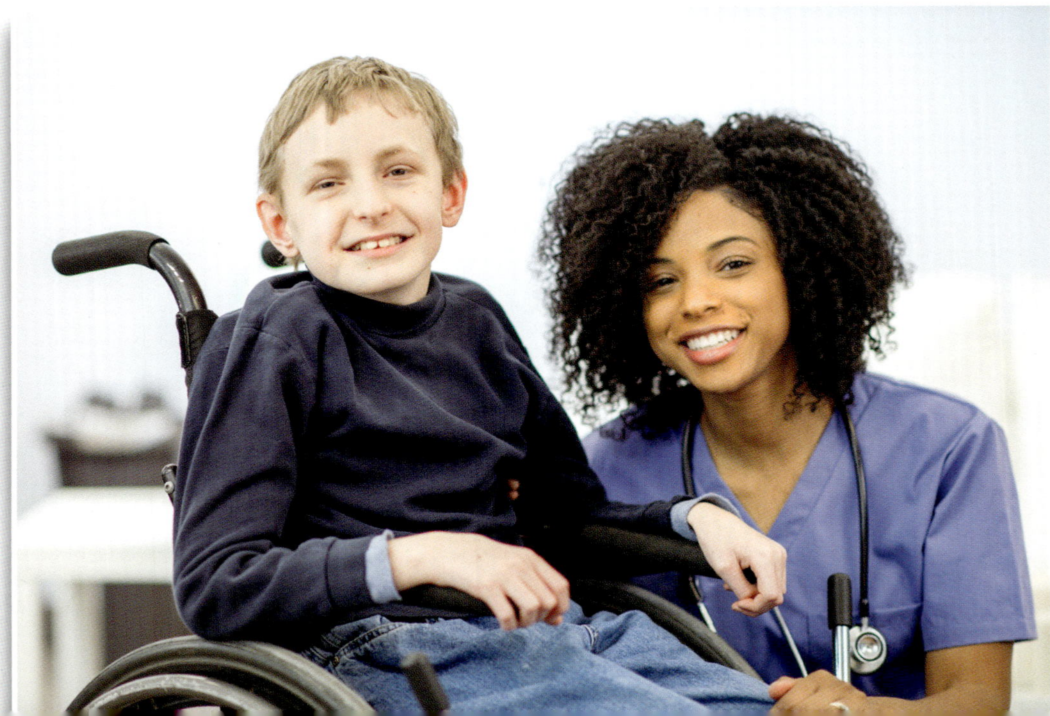

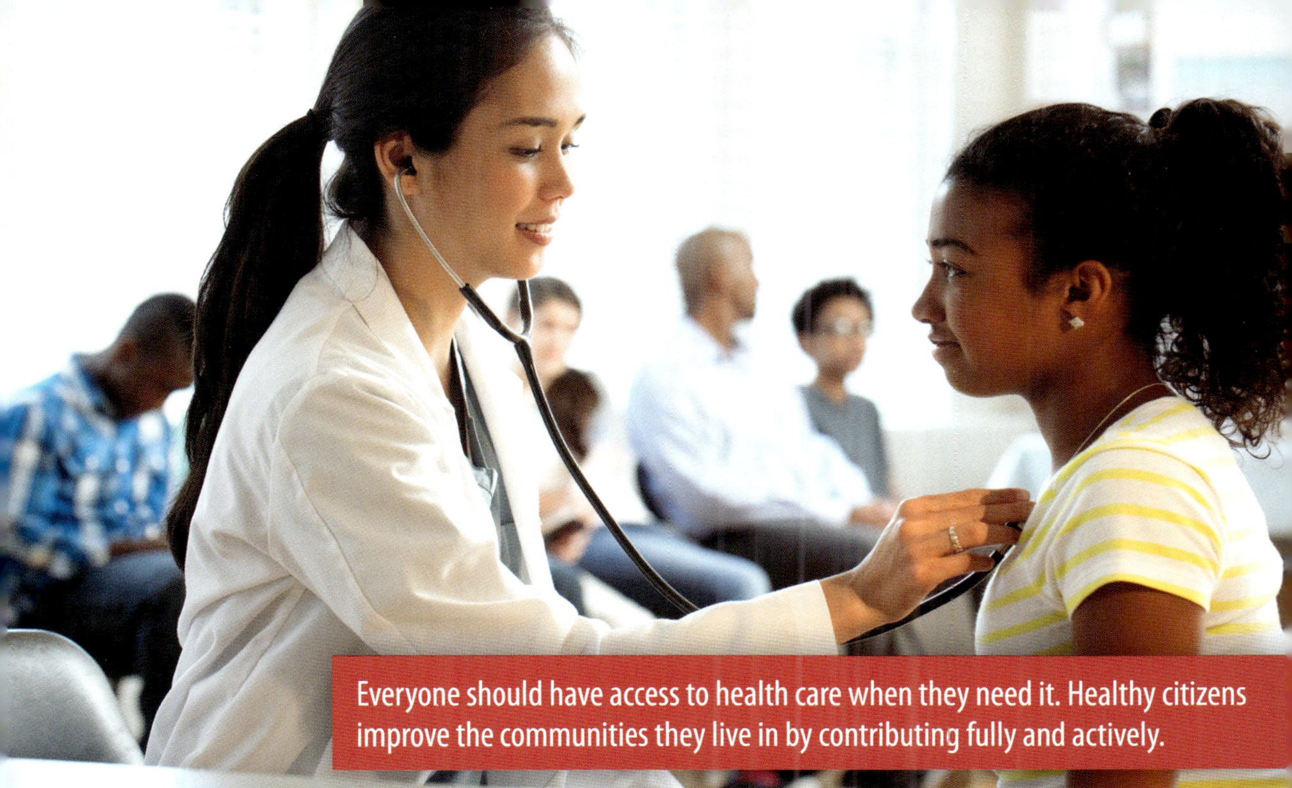

Everyone should have access to health care when they need it. Healthy citizens improve the communities they live in by contributing fully and actively.

The fields of medicine and public health are designed to meet that challenge. The medical field focuses on detecting and treating diseases using science and technology. Public health workers aim to prevent disease and prolong life by researching causes, tracking illness and injury, and providing education. Working together, people in these fields can improve life for people around the world.

In 2015, the United Nations (UN) adopted a number of goals to boost health and well-being. The UN's goal is to reach its targets for physical health by 2030. These goals include stopping dangerous communicable diseases from spreading, preventing and treating noncommunicable diseases, reducing environmental pollution, providing better care for mothers and young children, and offering universal health coverage so everyone has access to lifesaving medicines and care. These goals draw attention to some of the greatest barriers to maintaining good physical health today.

CHAPTER TWO

A HISTORY OF DISEASE AND MEDICINE

From ancient to modern times, the spread of disease, a lack of healthy food, and a wide range of environmental factors have threatened health. However, ideas about health and the treatment of illnesses have changed over time. Scientific theories and technologies have revolutionized our understanding of disease and medicine.

Disease and illness have always been part of human life. When hunter-gatherers settled into agricultural lifestyles, diseases became more common. Illnesses spread between humans and the animals they domesticated for food. Some agricultural societies relied on only a few crops for food, and their diets were missing key nutrients. As human settlements grew, diseases passed more easily between people. These groups also faced the challenges of finding clean drinking water and disposing safely of wastes.

Ancient peoples looked to myths, religious ideas, and superstitions to account for diseases. Many religions enforced rules about cleanliness and sanitation for spiritual reasons. These rules also worked to prevent disease. An ancient Greek doctor named Hippocrates studied disease in a more scientific way in the fifth or fourth century BC. He suggested that disease resulted from imbalances in the body or problems in the environment. Hippocrates made a distinction between what we now called epidemic diseases and endemic diseases. Epidemic diseases spread quickly and in large numbers. Endemic diseases are limited to a specific environment. These terms helped people think in new ways about how diseases came about, and they're still used today.

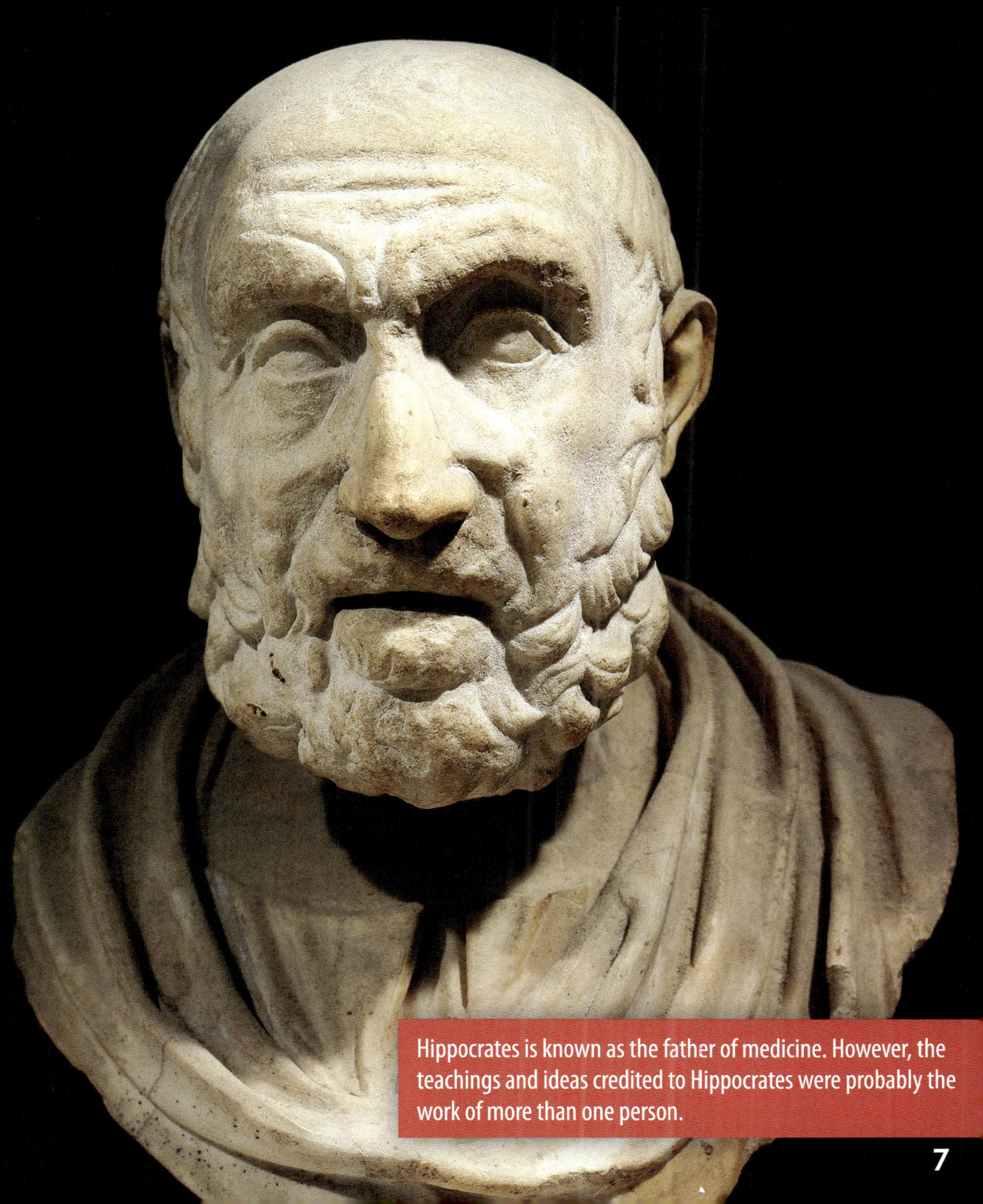

Hippocrates is known as the father of medicine. However, the teachings and ideas credited to Hippocrates were probably the work of more than one person.

In the Middle Ages, large populations and increasingly packed cities led to the spread of disease. Contagious diseases swept around the world throughout this period, starting with the plague, which hit Constantinople in AD 542. Epidemics of diseases called leprosy, smallpox, and tuberculosis were also common. The greatest tool in combating large epidemics was isolating infected people, or setting them apart from others.

After the Black Death ravaged Europe in the 1300s, countries introduced quarantines to keep travelers and merchants from spreading the disease. A quarantine is a period of time in which a person possibly exposed to a disease is isolated. They're free to go after a time if it's clear they haven't been infected.

Many of the diseases of the Middle Ages were caused by poor sanitation. The accumulation of garbage and waste in cities attracted rats, which helped spread diseases such as the plague. Diseases also spread quickly between people in crowded living conditions.

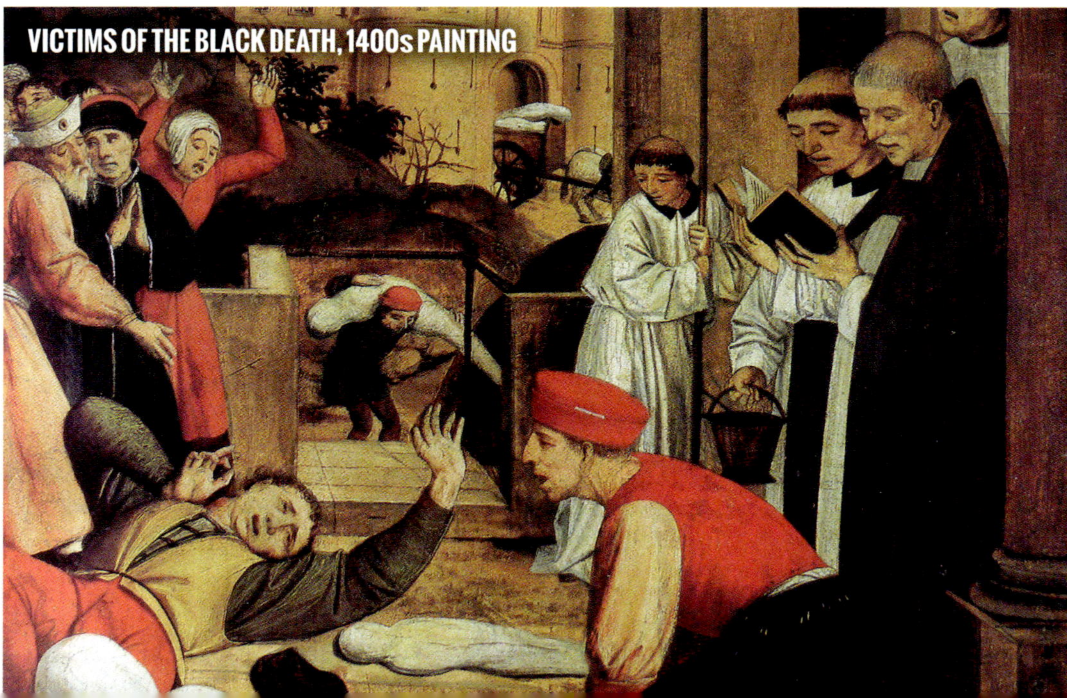

VICTIMS OF THE BLACK DEATH, 1400s PAINTING

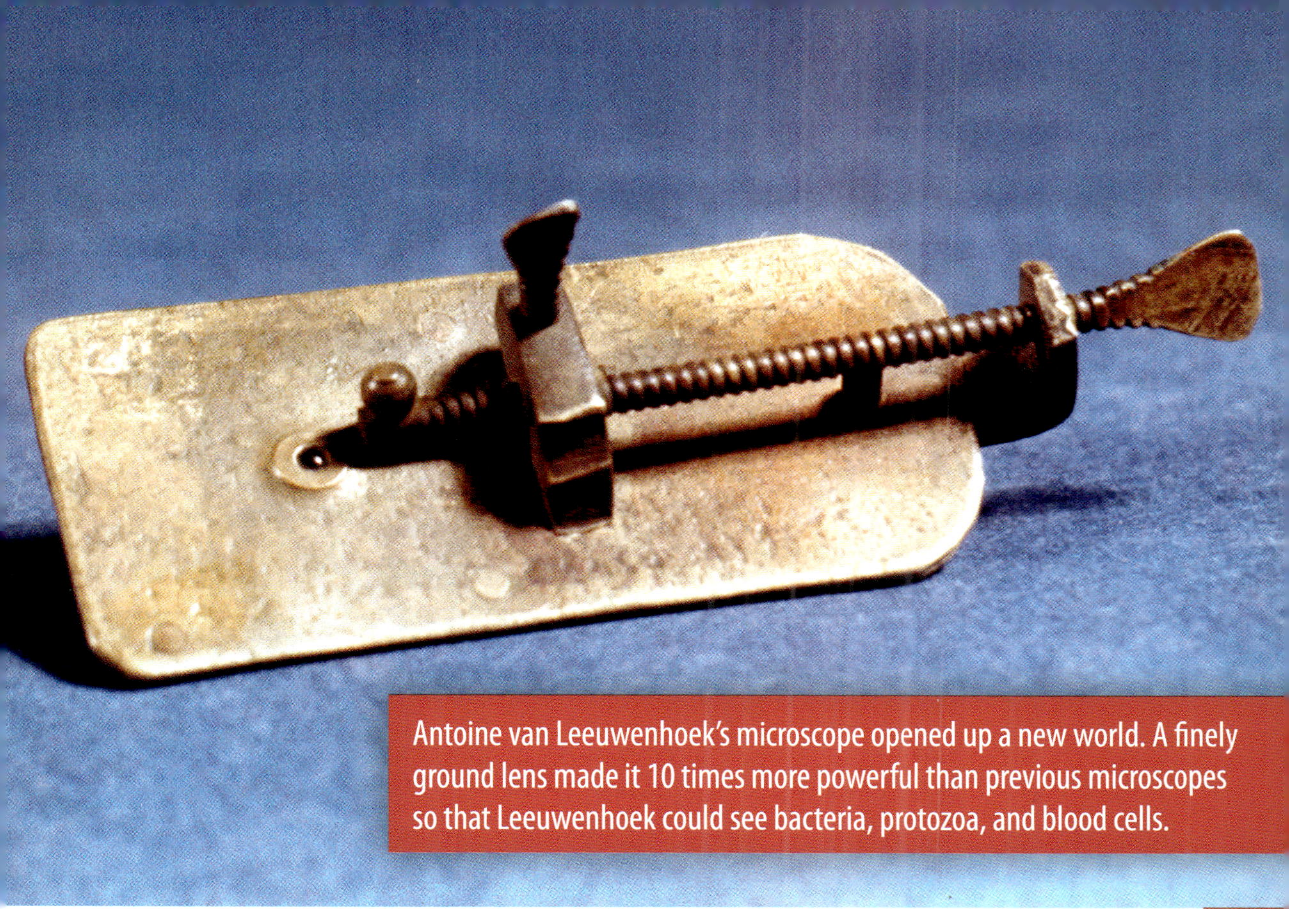

Antoine van Leeuwenhoek's microscope opened up a new world. A finely ground lens made it 10 times more powerful than previous microscopes so that Leeuwenhoek could see bacteria, protozoa, and blood cells.

Technological and scientific advances supported a greater understanding of how diseases spread. Scientist Antoine van Leeuwenhoek's improvements on the microscope allowed him to view bacteria for the first time in the 1670s. This was a step in understanding how microscopic organisms like bacteria could cause disease.

In the Age of Enlightenment (early 18th century), a radical idea took root. Philosophers taught that promoting health was the responsibility of good governments. Not only would this benefit individuals, healthy citizens would add to the economic success of society as a whole. The idea that improvements in health would lead to improvements in society was one of the founding principles of public health.

In 1750, the population of Europe boomed and the need for health care increased. People established hospitals across Europe and North America in the 18th and 19th centuries. Besides serving the sick, these hospitals also became centers of medical study and training.

At the same time, the Industrial Revolution was changing health, especially for poor workers. Death rates rose as dangerous work conditions threatened lives and disease spread through crammed and filthy cities. Reformers promoted changes for safe housing and the welfare of workers. Health education also targeted unsanitary practices and worked to prevent diseases before they happened. Civic engineers proposed many solutions, including waste disposal, for sanitary concerns.

Meanwhile, doctors and scientists were making important discoveries by observing and recording information about health problems and treatments. Sanitation was a major concern. Preventing and treating epidemics of diseases such as smallpox, yellow fever, typhoid, typhus, and cholera were also priorities. With new science and data from these studies, the 20th century witnessed advances in vaccination, regulations for safer workplaces, and the introduction of different medicines and treatments.

People have made extraordinary advances in medicine, but many worldwide health challenges persist. Providing lifesaving vaccinations can minimize the threat of many communicable diseases. Preventing the spread of the diseases AIDS, malaria, and tuberculosis are other health goals. Malnutrition, or poor nutrition, is a major concern around the world, as are the dangers of noncommunicable illnesses such as cancer and heart disease. Controlling environmental factors and pollution is also necessary. Overall, global health can be improved by meeting these goals and creating effective health-care systems.

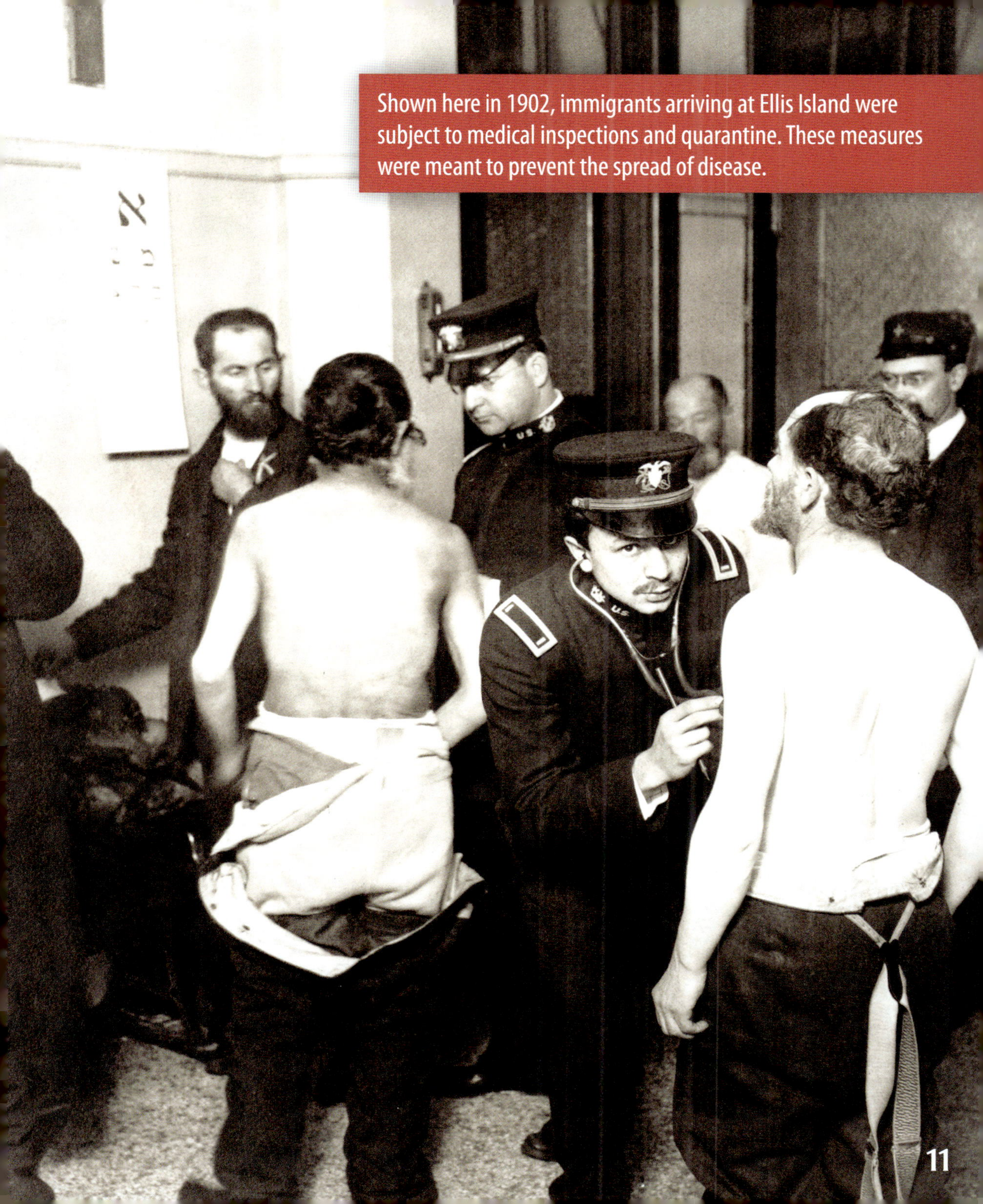

Shown here in 1902, immigrants arriving at Ellis Island were subject to medical inspections and quarantine. These measures were meant to prevent the spread of disease.

CHAPTER THREE

PREVENTION THROUGH VACCINATION

Vaccination is one of the most powerful tools available for fighting contagious diseases and improving public health. A particular vaccination provides limited exposure to specific germs. These are the same germs that cause a disease, but they're weakened so the body can fight them and build an immunity to the disease. If the body encounters a stronger form of the disease later, it likely won't be infected.

People used early forms of vaccination in ancient Chinese and Indian medicine to prevent smallpox, a disease that caused a dangerous fever and rash. English physician Edward Jenner further developed these techniques in 1796 and created a highly effective smallpox vaccination method. Smallpox vaccination continued over the next few centuries, and by 1979, the disease was officially eradicated, or eliminated.

Another great vaccination breakthrough occurred in 1955, when the American Scientist Jonas Salk perfected the polio vaccine. The polio virus often affects children and can lead to paralysis or death. Salk's vaccine provided protection from the disease and prevented widespread outbreaks.

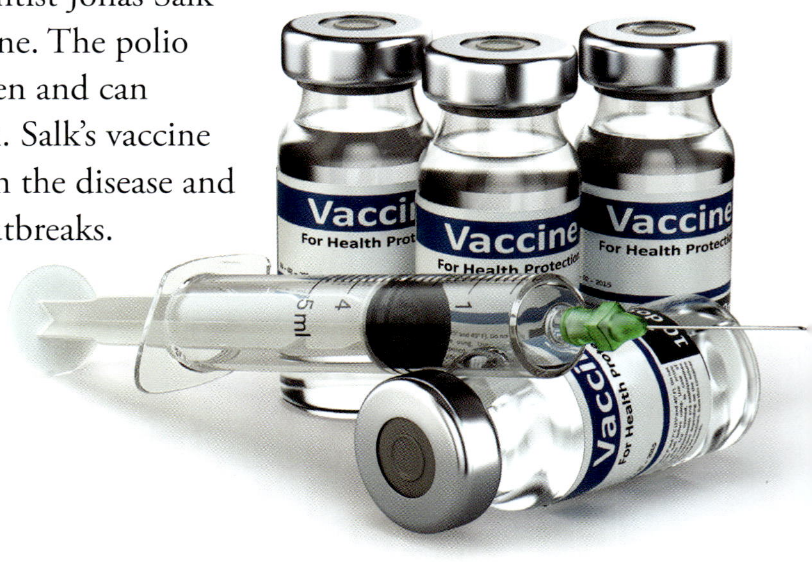

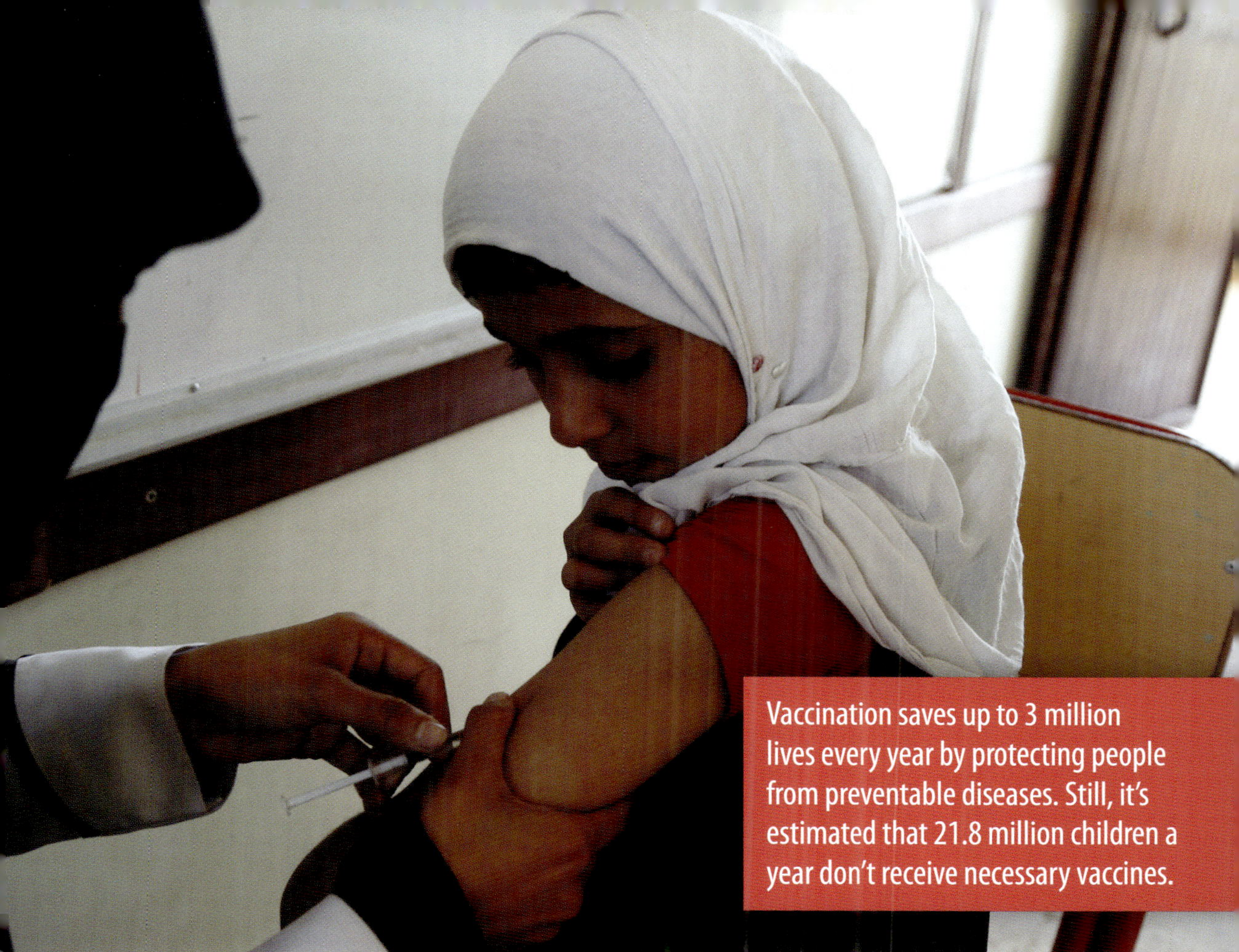

Vaccination saves up to 3 million lives every year by protecting people from preventable diseases. Still, it's estimated that 21.8 million children a year don't receive necessary vaccines.

World health workers also provide vaccinations against the diseases diphtheria, tetanus, pertussis, measles, mumps, and rubella. Like polio, these diseases commonly affect children. Measles is currently a severe risk for unvaccinated children. Over 300 children die from measles every day. Making vaccination easy and available around the world can greatly reduce illness and death in children under age five.

In recent years, there has been a growing anti-vaccination movement in the United States. Debunking common misconceptions about immunization and raising awareness about the serious risks of foregoing vaccinations will help ensure a safer, healthier future for all.

CHAPTER FOUR

COMMUNICABLE DISEASES

Although vaccinations are effective in preventing some communicable diseases, others, such as HIV/AIDS, require additional methods. The human immunodeficiency virus (HIV) attacks the immune system so a person can't fight off infections. If left untreated, HIV leads to acquired immunodeficiency syndrome (AIDS). This is the advanced stage of the virus, when many different infections weaken the body and can lead to death.

HIV can be transmitted through contact with body fluids. It's often passed between sexual partners. Infected mothers can transfer the disease to their children during pregnancy, childbirth, or breastfeeding. It can also be passed through blood. This sometimes occurs through shared and contaminated needles or medical equipment.

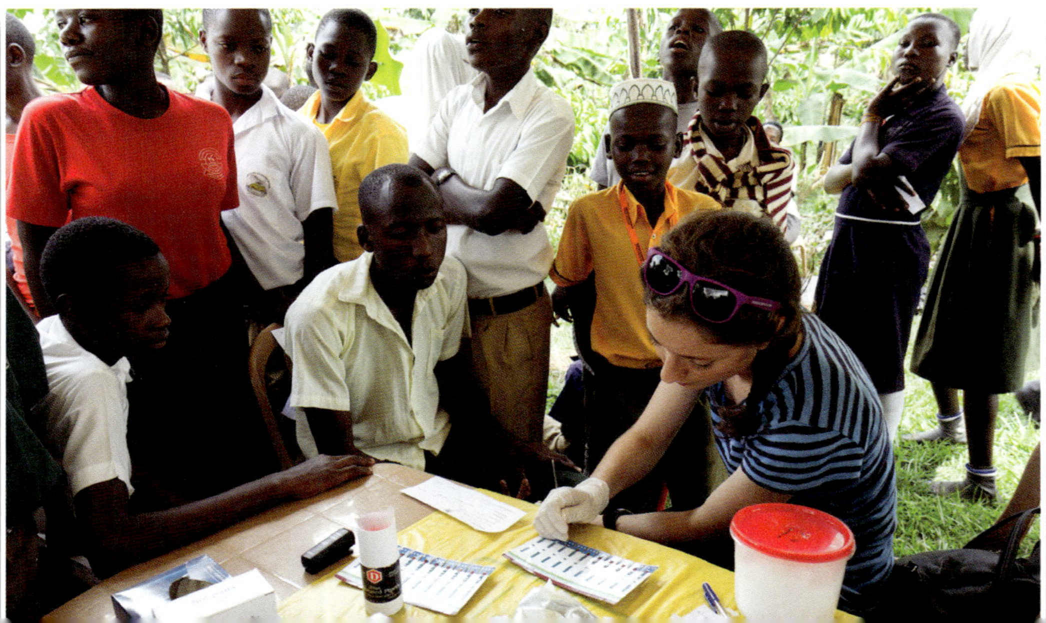

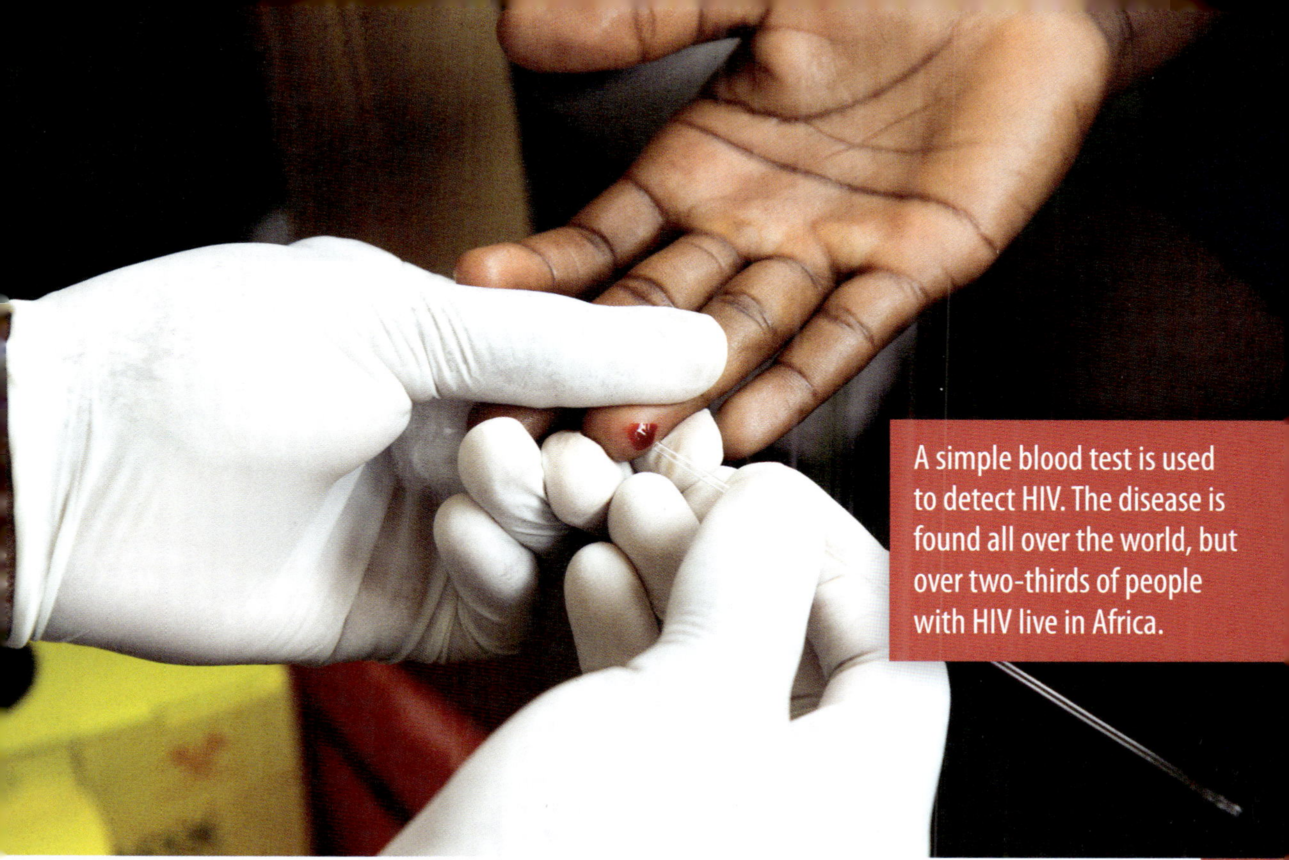

A simple blood test is used to detect HIV. The disease is found all over the world, but over two-thirds of people with HIV live in Africa.

Since it was first identified in 1983, HIV has been difficult to control. So far, 32 million people have died as a result. But today, medications can stop HIV from progressing to AIDS. They can even limit the virus in the body until it can't be passed on to other people. Other medicines keep mothers from passing HIV to their infants. There's still no cure for HIV, but the right medications can keep the disease in check.

Education plays an important role in preventing HIV. Providing information about how to have safe and protected sex is a key feature of HIV education. Preventing AIDS by getting tested and treated for HIV is another element. Today, about 37.9 million people have HIV. With the right treatment and education, new cases can be avoided and people with the disease can live longer and healthier lives.

Other communicable diseases that are major threats around the world are tuberculosis, malaria, and hepatitis. Tuberculosis is a top cause of death. It claimed 1.5 million lives in 2018. The disease is found everywhere, but more than 95 percent of new cases are in developing countries. In addition, many people with HIV become infected with tuberculosis.

Tuberculosis is caused by bacteria passed through the air when an infected person coughs, sneezes, or spits. The bacteria can infect the lungs. However, tuberculosis can be prevented with vaccination and cured with medication. Providing access to diagnosis and treatment, especially in developing countries, is very important.

Similarly, malaria mostly affects people in developing countries, especially in Africa. Mosquito bites pass parasites to people. Malaria produces a fever that can quickly become deadly. There were 228 million cases and 405,000 deaths from malaria in 2018. The disease is most deadly in infants and children under five years old. People can prevent malaria with the use of special mosquito nets at night and sprays in homes.

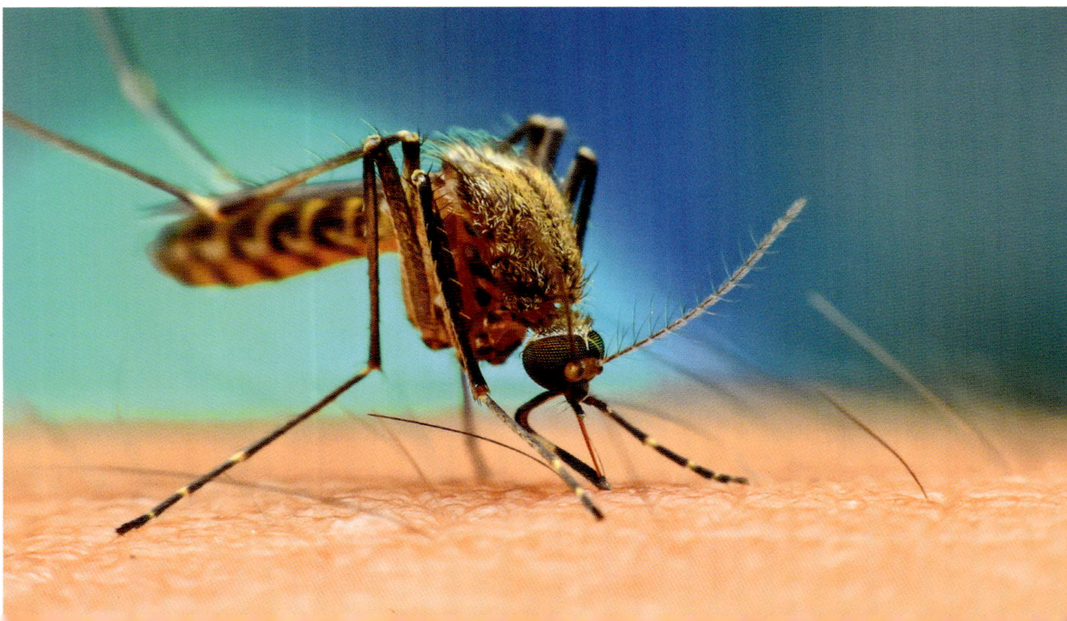

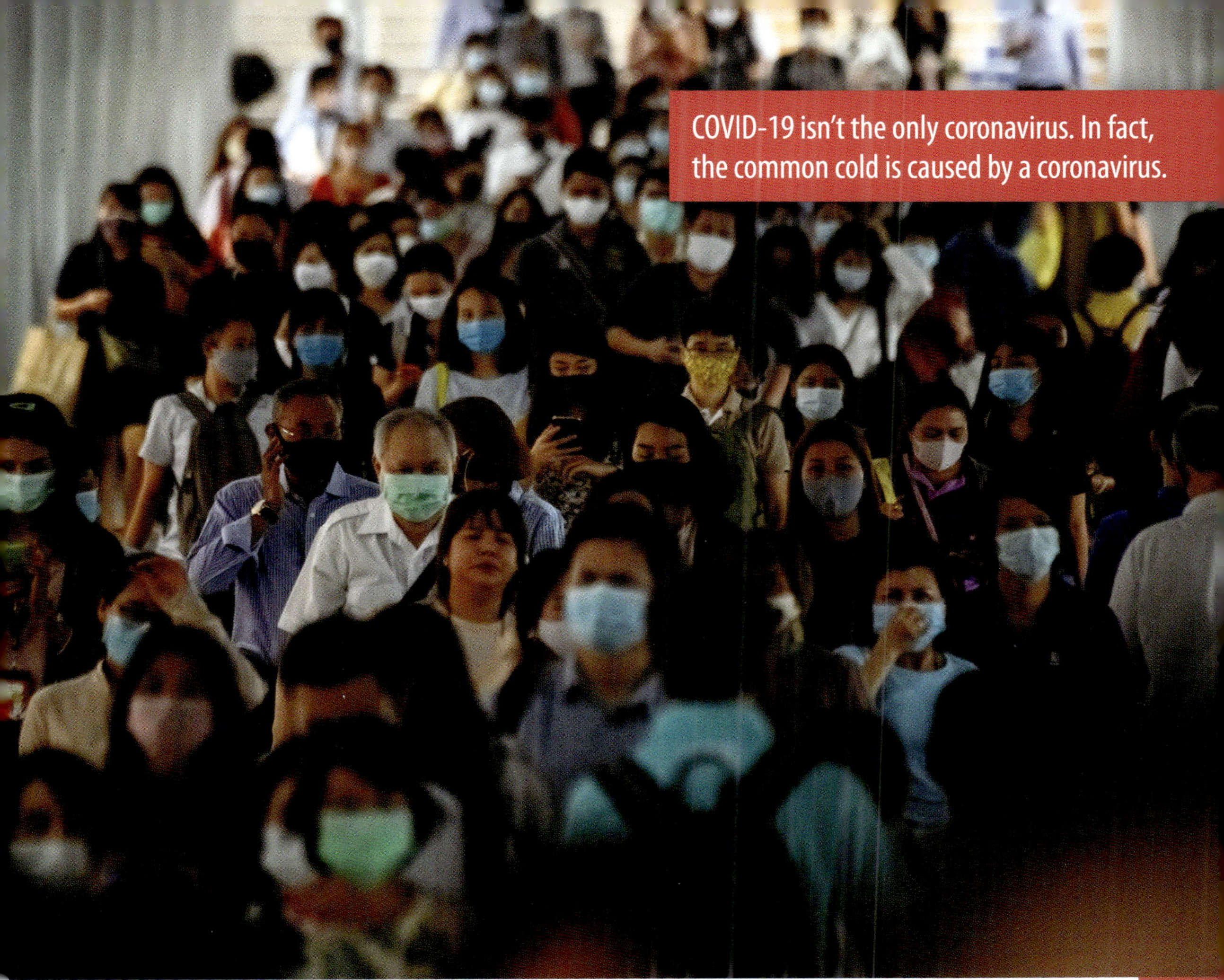

COVID-19 isn't the only coronavirus. In fact, the common cold is caused by a coronavirus.

Early in 2020, a new illness spread throughout the world. COVID-19 (coronavirus disease 2019) became an epidemic in China in early 2020, but soon after, it became a pandemic affecting people all over the world. By October 2020, more than 36 million people had fallen ill with the disease, and more than 1 million people had died.

COVID-19 is a virus that can be spread to others in the form of tiny droplets when people cough or sneeze. Scientists around the world urged people to wear masks and practice social distancing, but the pandemic lasted for many months.

CHAPTER FIVE

NONCOMMUNICABLE DISEASES

In addition to communicable diseases, many noncommunicable diseases threaten physical health around the world. The most common of these are diabetes, cardiovascular diseases, and cancer, which account for over 70 percent of deaths. These diseases are often linked to poverty. They can affect people at any age and increase the chance of early death.

Lifestyle, genetics, and environmental conditions place some people at higher risk for some noncommunicable diseases. Habits like tobacco and alcohol use, poor diet, and lack of physical activity are important factors. Prevention for noncommunicable diseases focuses on changing these habits.

Diabetes is related to insulin, a hormone that regulates blood sugar. In type I diabetes, the body doesn't make enough insulin. In type II diabetes, the body isn't able to use insulin well. Type II is more common, and it sometimes results from having extra weight and a lack of exercise. In 2019, 463 million adults had diabetes.

Diseases that affect the heart and blood vessels are called cardiovascular diseases. They can lead to heart attack and stroke, and they're the number one cause of death in the world. Many cardiovascular diseases can be prevented with a healthy lifestyle.

Cancer describes a wide range of diseases that lead to abnormal cell growth in different organs and tissues in the body. Cancer is difficult and expensive to treat, and it's the second most common cause of death in the world. Prevention, early detection, and treatment of noncommunicable diabetes, cardiovascular disease, and cancer are global goals.

When he was in the eighth grade, Rishab Jain developed new software to help treat pancreatic cancer. Jain's technology allows doctors to more accurately locate the pancreas during radiation treatments.

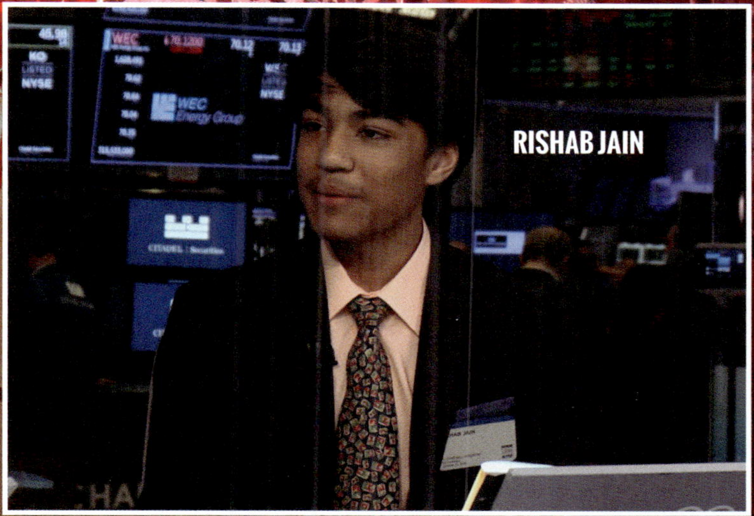

CHAPTER SIX

RISKS FROM POLLUTION

Although many noncommunicable diseases are related to lifestyle, environmental factors also matter. Water and soil pollution pose health challenges around the world, but air pollution is the most widespread. It's responsible for 7 million deaths a year, and it leads to one-third of deaths from stroke, lung cancer, and heart disease. It also causes and worsens respiratory infections and the condition called asthma.

Burning fossil fuels, which releases particles and gases into the air, creates air pollution. "Particulate matter" refers to tiny particles that people breathe into the lungs from polluted air. Some particles are so small they can pass from the lungs into the bloodstream. Particulate matter impairs the lungs, brain, and heart.

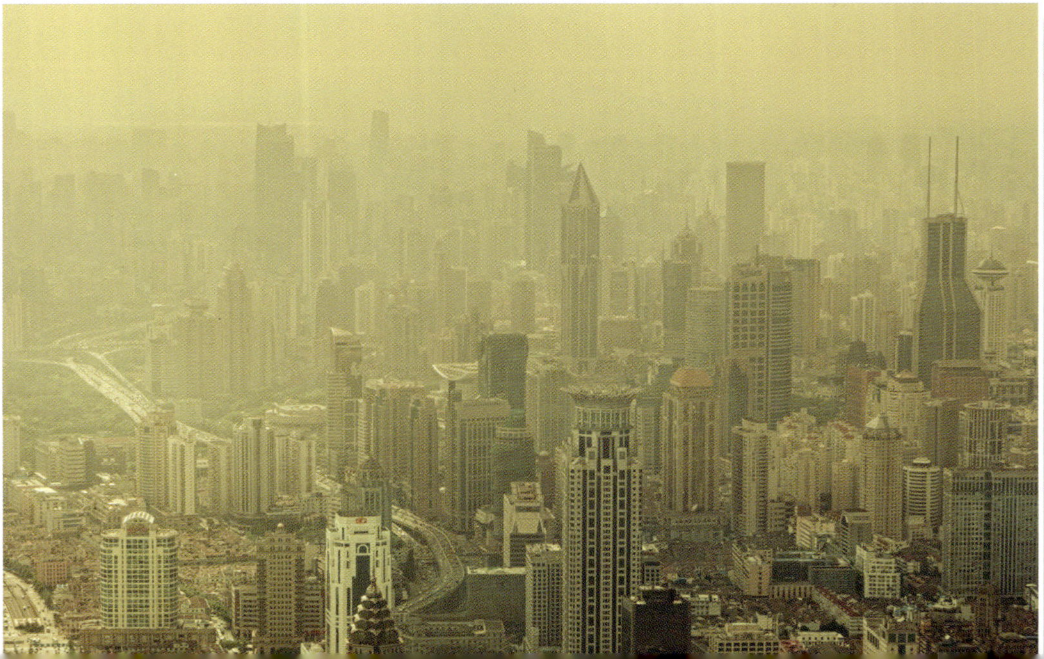

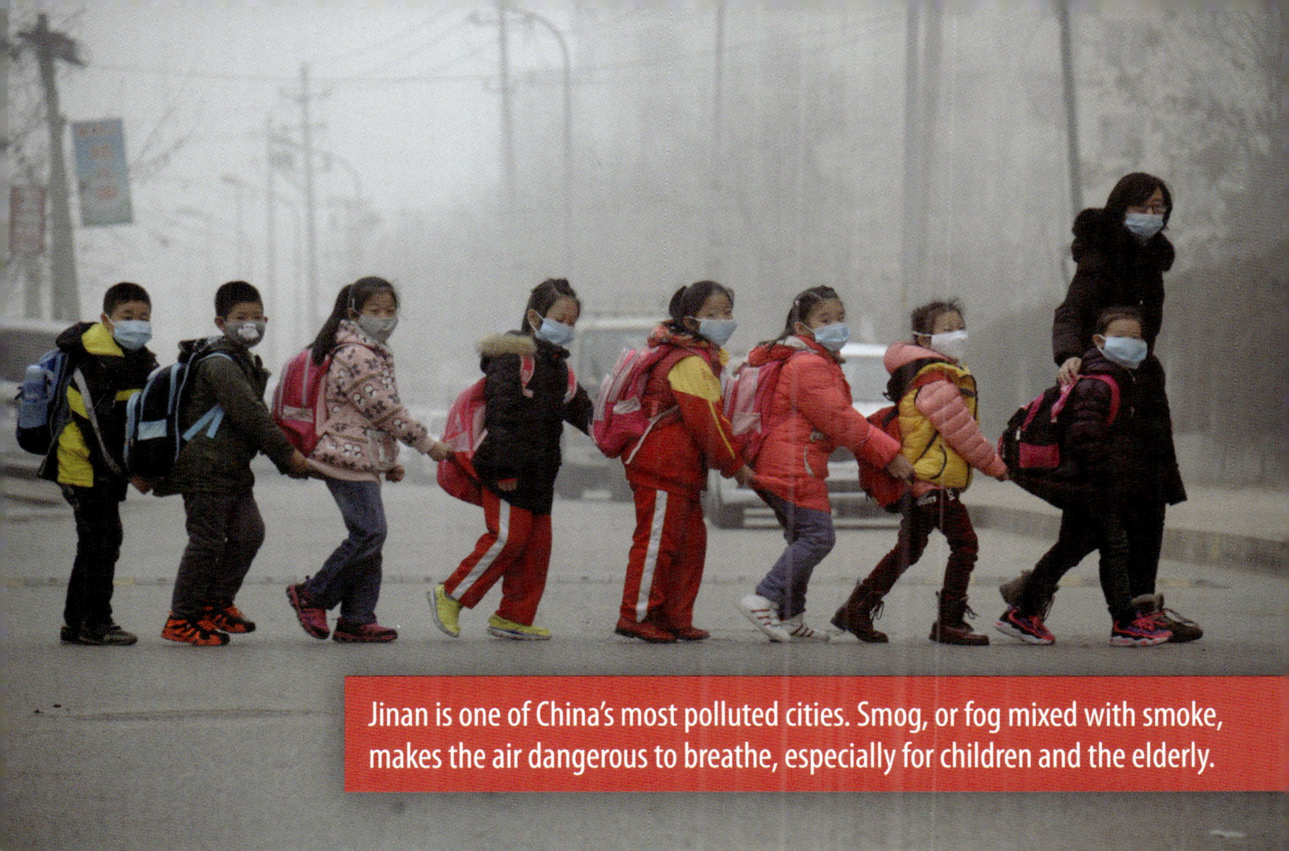

Jinan is one of China's most polluted cities. Smog, or fog mixed with smoke, makes the air dangerous to breathe, especially for children and the elderly.

Ambient air pollution happens outdoors and leads to 4.2 million deaths a year. It results from fumes and toxins created by vehicles, industries, and activities that burn wastes or fossil fuels. Roughly 90 percent of people sometimes breathe in air that's highly polluted.

Household air pollution mainly affects the developing world, where burning wood or coal at home is more common. These cooking, heating, and lighting practices produce smoke and particulate matter. Household air pollution causes 3.8 million deaths every year. It's chiefly harmful to women and children who spend more time at home.

The best way to reduce air pollution is to commit to clean and renewable, or able to be replaced, energy sources. Burning fossil fuels has caused a climate crisis and polluted air to unsafe levels. Efforts to solve climate change and air pollution go hand in hand.

CHAPTER SEVEN

GOOD NUTRITION

The World Health Organization (WHO) has called malnutrition one of the greatest challenges to world health. This problem is present in every country. Without intervention, three different types of malnutrition can lead to other illnesses, disabilities, or death.

One form of malnutrition is undernutrition. This occurs when a person doesn't have enough food to thrive. Children, who need healthy food to grow and develop, are especially vulnerable. Undernutrition weakens the body, making it harder to fight off other illnesses. As a result, about 45 percent of deaths in children under five years old are related to undernutrition. About 462 million adults are also undernourished.

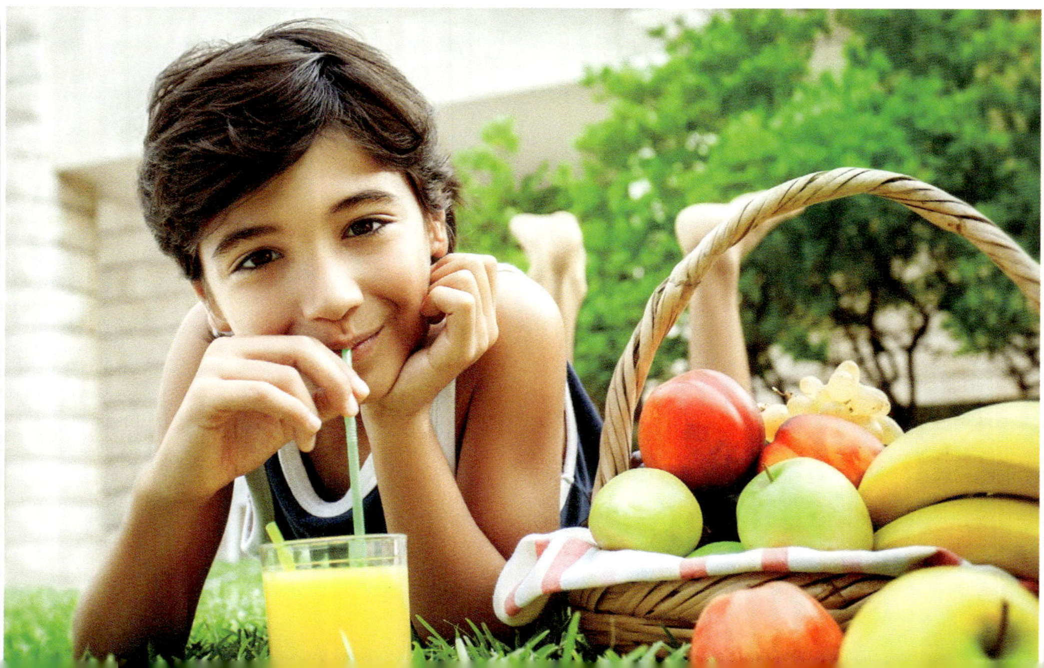

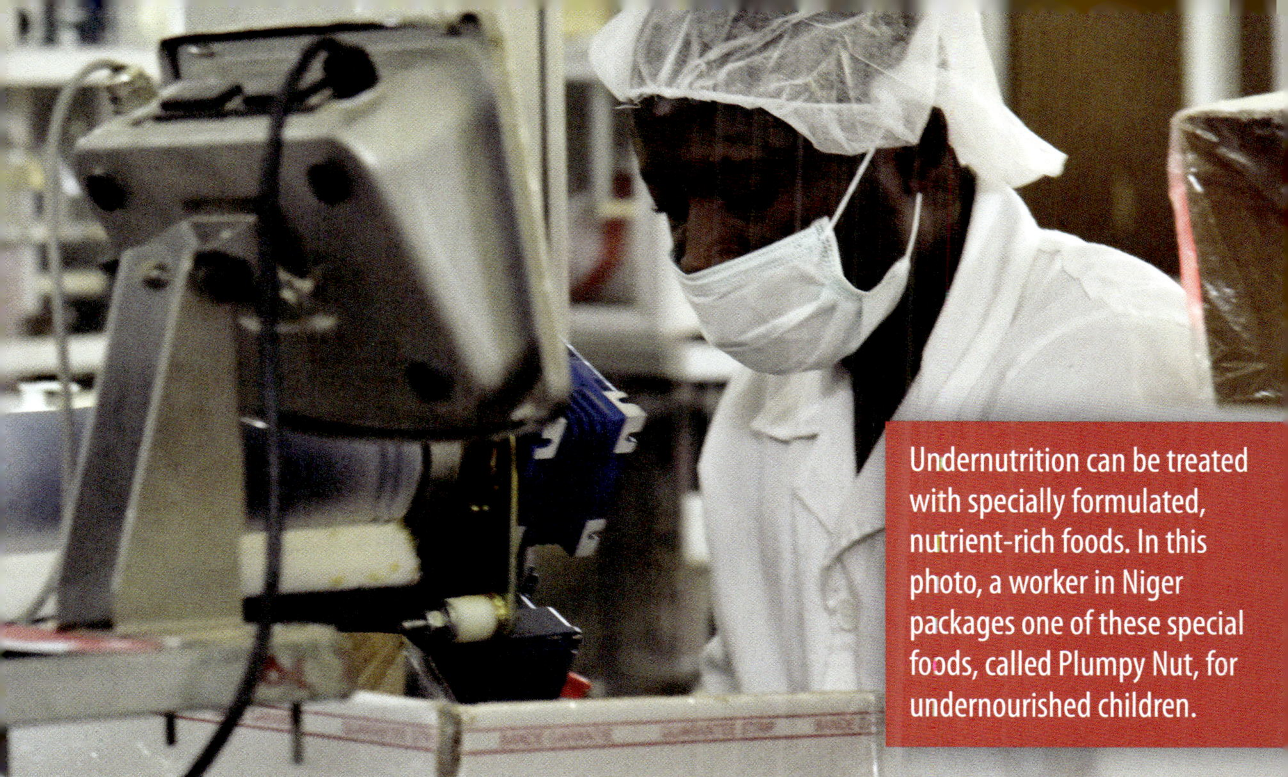

Undernutrition can be treated with specially formulated, nutrient-rich foods. In this photo, a worker in Niger packages one of these special foods, called Plumpy Nut, for undernourished children.

Another type of malnutrition develops when specific vitamins or minerals are missing from the diet. This is called a micronutrient deficiency, and it can also lead to poor health. Half a billion women around the world suffer from a condition called anemia from low iron intake. This can also put their children at risk if they're pregnant, but it can be treated with iron supplements.

The conditions of being overweight or obese make up the third category of malnutrition. Roughly 2.3 billion people are overweight or obese, including 38 million children under five. The conditions can lead to noncommunicable diseases. Fortunately, a balanced diet and exercise help.

In many places, the three different forms of malnutrition exist side by side. Solutions focus on education about healthy nutrition and food aid to vulnerable populations. Rethinking food systems to combat climate change is also important in areas where extreme weather conditions affect crops.

CHAPTER EIGHT

REPRODUCTIVE HEALTH

Reproductive health is concerned with sexual health and the ability to reproduce as desired. Many reproductive health initiatives deal with the health of mothers and their babies. Today's reproductive medicine is highly advanced with effective tools. Still, many people don't have access to these necessary reproductive health services.

Honest sex education and the availability of contraception are vital components of reproductive health. Both tools can prevent sexually transmitted diseases (STDs) and unintentional pregnancies. Making modern contraception accessible could help the millions of women who have unwanted pregnancies. Preventing violence against women is another way to ensure that pregnancies only occur when they're desired.

This is especially important since pregnancy and childbirth often have tragic consequences. In 2017, 295,000 women died as a result of childbirth. About 2.6 million babies died in or shortly before childbirth, and another 2.6 million died within the first 28 days of life. The health of mothers and of infants is closely linked, and they both need to be treated by skilled providers before, during, and after birth.

Most mother or infant deaths are preventable. We have the knowledge, medicine, and technology to make childbirth safe. Unfortunately, many people in developing countries can't reach trained health-care providers. They may live in remote areas without care facilities. In response, national and international organizations have pushed for better reproductive care. Most regions of the world have reduced the number of deaths connected with childbirth since 2000.

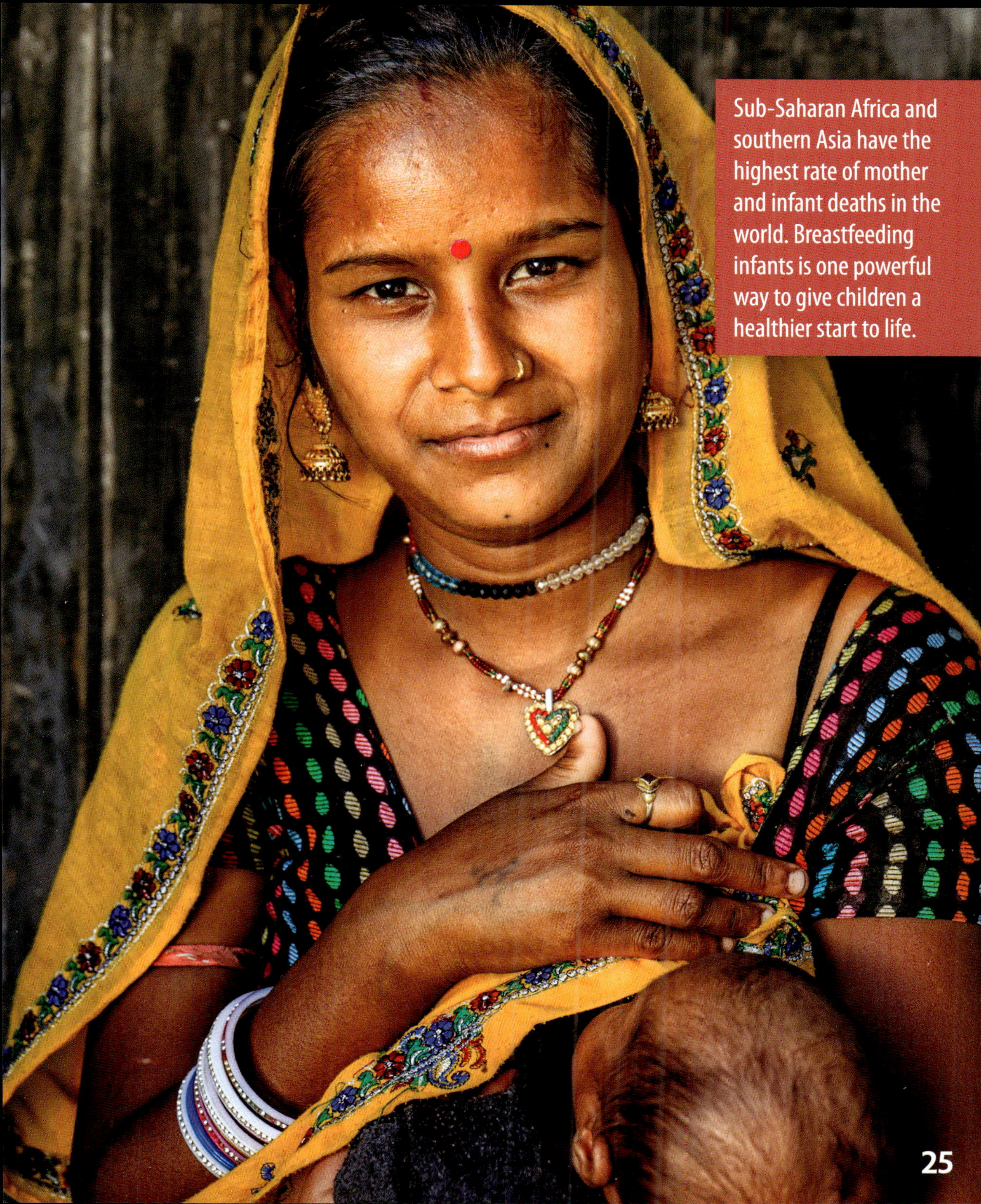

Sub-Saharan Africa and southern Asia have the highest rate of mother and infant deaths in the world. Breastfeeding infants is one powerful way to give children a healthier start to life.

CHAPTER NINE

UNIVERSAL HEALTH COVERAGE

Part of promoting physical health for all is building up accessible and effective health-care systems. Universal health coverage is the only way to ensure that all people receive services to promote health and prevent and treat problems. Currently, 1 billion people don't have basic health care.

It's important that people of all income levels have opportunities to improve their health through quality care without fear of financial harm. Health is a human right, and no one should be denied necessary medications and treatments because they can't pay for them. Countries and governments must find the best way to provide for the health needs of their citizens. International organizations can offer resources to the poorest countries as they establish quality health systems.

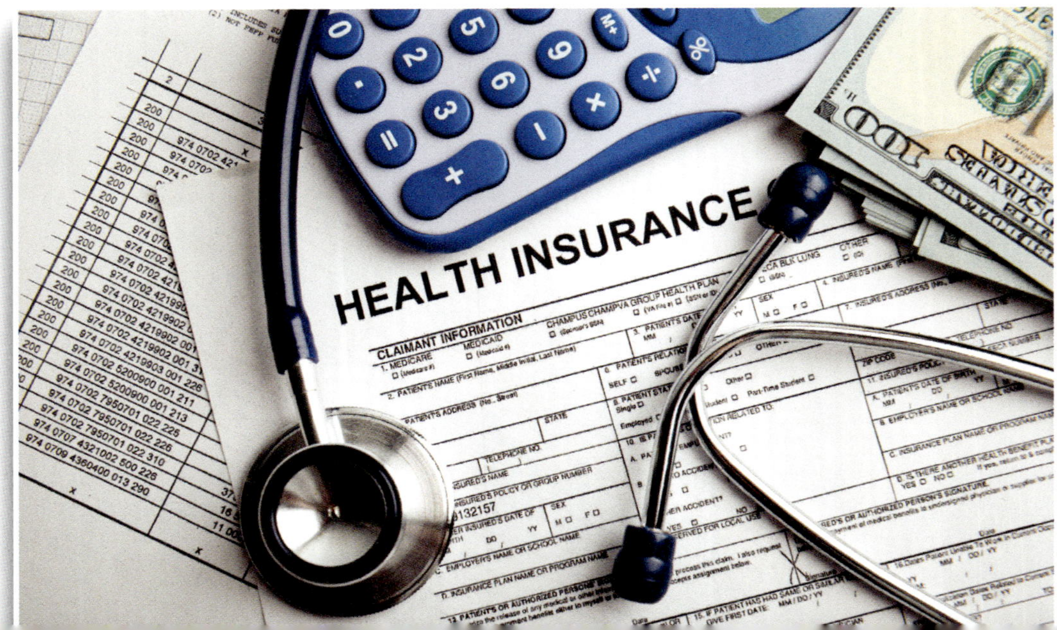

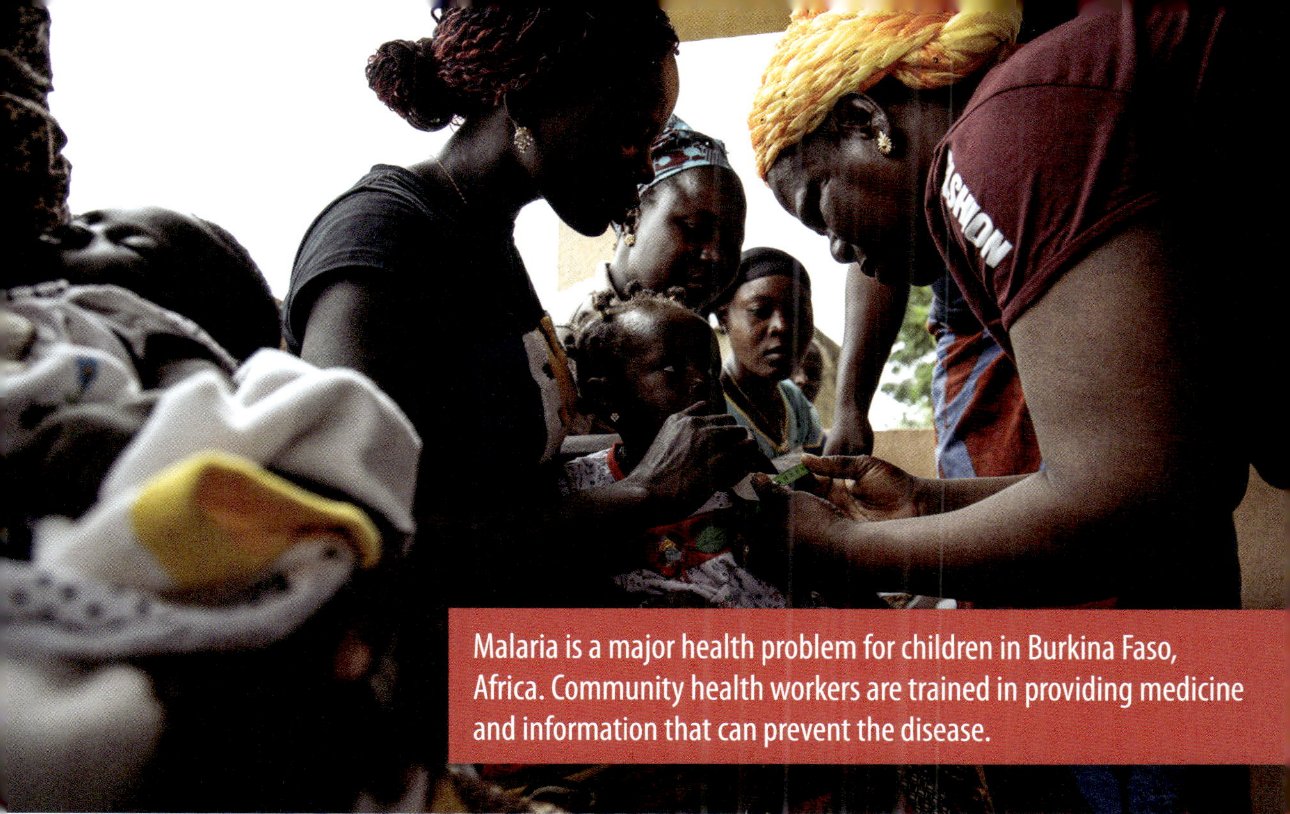

Malaria is a major health problem for children in Burkina Faso, Africa. Community health workers are trained in providing medicine and information that can prevent the disease.

Offering strong primary care services is one of the best methods for improving health around the world. Primary care nurses and doctors offer basic health services rather than specialized treatments. They play a key role in promoting well-being, preventing illness, and detecting health problems early.

In developing countries, supporting community health workers is a major tool for providing health care to people in remote locations. These caregivers are a critical access point in receiving health services. They're community members who've been trained to offer a certain range of health services. These might include providing vaccinations, medicines, and life-saving skills.

In the United States, about 44 million people have no health insurance. Developing smarter, fairer, and more effective health systems everywhere should be a global goal.

CHAPTER TEN

IMPROVING CARE WITH TECHNOLOGY

Technology has made many great advances of modern medicine possible. Doctors and scientists have a deeper and more accurate understanding of physical health and disease than ever before. Medical technology has been specially developed to detect diseases, find and perfect treatments, and keep an eye on health. New technologies also have a role in making health-care services more accessible to people around the world.

Fitness trackers and apps encourage people to take an active role in observing their own health and activity. Over 160,000 health-related apps have been designed to track behaviors such as food and water intake, exercise, sleep, and use of medications. These apps may have a significant effect in preventing diabetes and heart disease. Many apps are also designed to educate and support pregnant mothers before, during, and after childbirth with information and reminders.

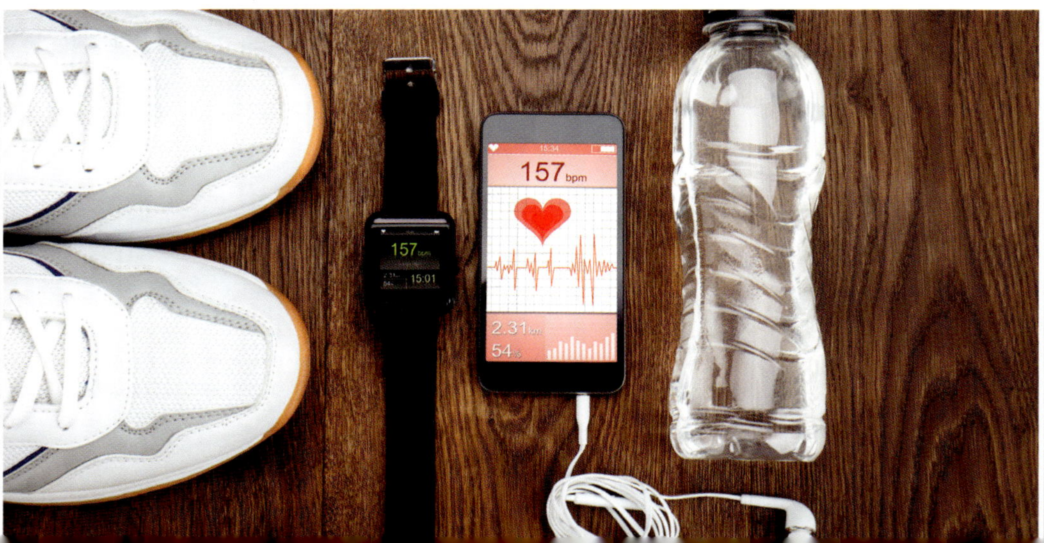

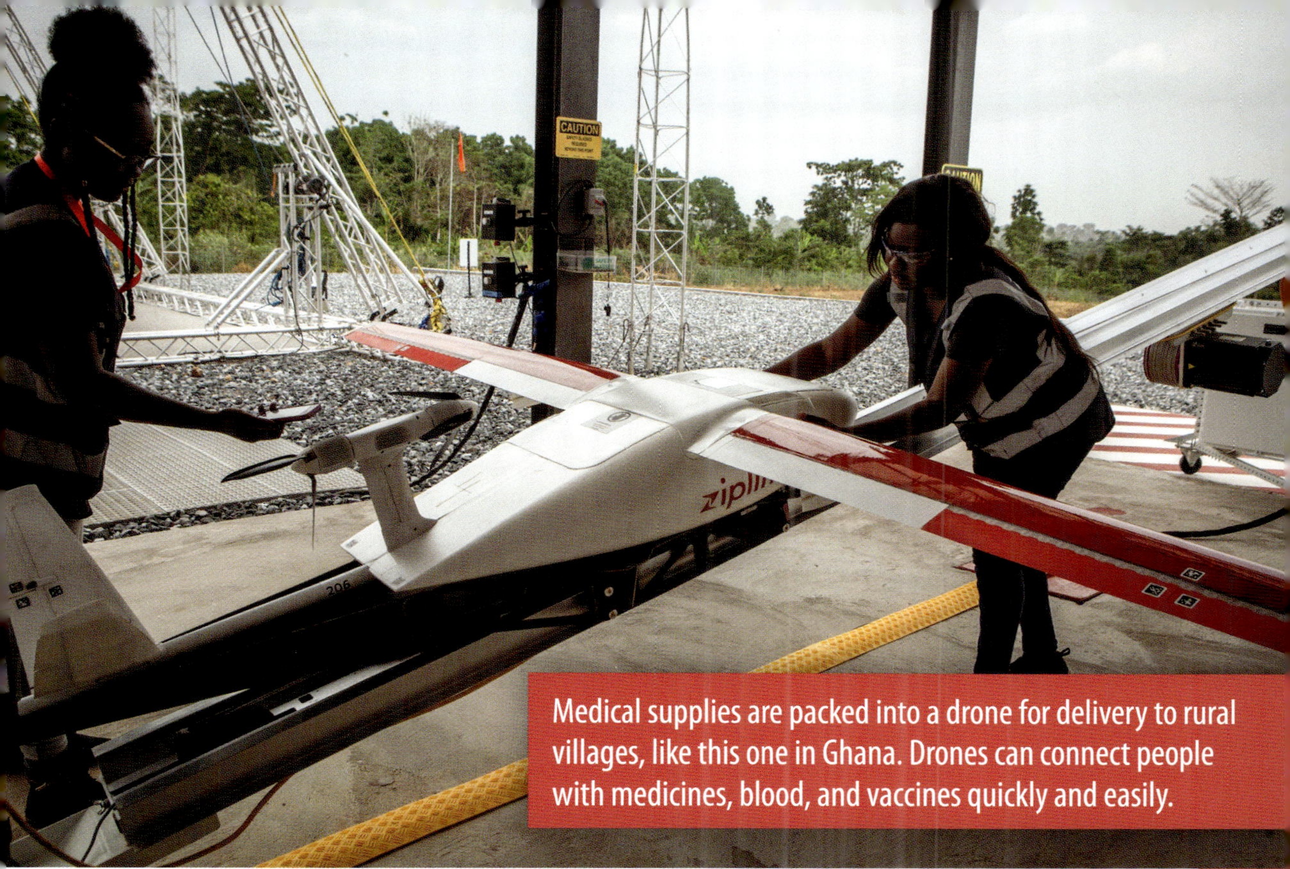

Medical supplies are packed into a drone for delivery to rural villages, like this one in Ghana. Drones can connect people with medicines, blood, and vaccines quickly and easily.

Mobile technologies such as video calling can extend medical services to isolated populations. In rural Bangladesh, a program called Teledaktar provides virtual doctor appointments. Operators who are trained to use some health-screening tools set up a laptop that connects with a volunteer doctor elsewhere. Using video calling, the doctor can answer health questions, write prescriptions, diagnose problems, and refer patients to the nearest specialist who can help them.

From small, transportable imaging devices to 3-D printed prostheses, or artificial parts, engineers are constantly contributing to world health. Making new technologies available and affordable can make a difference in improving physical health for all. Developing technologies that are specially designed to support the most vulnerable people is key.

CHAPTER ELEVEN

ACTION FOR HEALTH

Improving physical health around the world is a large and complicated task, but everyone can contribute. Health care and governments are closely connected. You can take action by calling for government policies that promote health in your own country and in the world.

Young people have become strong advocates for new environmental standards. Climate change is linked to several key physical health issues, including nutrition and air pollution. You can join the campaign by taking part in protests that demand change. You can also make daily choices to use fewer fossil fuels in your home and community. Lessening climate change and air pollution will help everyone in the world breathe easier.

Another way to start working for global health is to choose an issue that's important to you. Nujeen Mustafa became a spokesperson for people with disabilities when she spoke out about her own experiences. Mustafa was born with cerebral palsy, a condition that made her unable to walk. When she was 16, Mustafa fled from Syria to escape conflict. She journeyed with her sister for 3,500 miles (5,632.7 km) to Germany, traveling by bus, train, boat, and land in her wheelchair. The difficulties along the way convinced Mustafa that people with disabilities needed special consideration as refugees. Since then, Mustafa has addressed world leaders and argued for the recognition and inclusion of people with disabilities when planning for emergencies. Mustafa's story shows that if you're passionate about an issue, your interests and experiences can inspire you to work for change.

GLOSSARY

advocate (AD-vuh-kuht) A person who argues for or supports a cause or policy.

contraception (kahn-truh-SEP-shuhn) Methods of birth control to prevent pregnancy.

crisis (KRY-suhs) An unstable or difficult situation.

domesticate (duh-MEH-stih-kayt) To breed and raise an animal for use by people.

drone (DROHN) A pilotless aircraft.

fossil fuel (FAH-suhl FYOOL) A fuel—such as coal, oil, or natural gas—that is formed in the earth from dead plants or animals.

genetics (juh-NEH-tiks) The genetic makeup of an organism.

intervention (in-tuhr-VEN-shuhn) The act of taking action about something to affect the outcome.

nutrient (NOO-tree-uhnt) Something taken in by a plant or animal that helps it grow and stay healthy.

nutrition (noo-TRIH-shuhn) The process of eating the right food to grow and be healthy.

parasite (PEHR-uh-syt) A living thing that lives in, on, or with another living thing and often harms it.

protozoa (proh-tuh-ZOH-uh) Microscopic organisms. The plural is protozoon.

radiation (ray-dee-AY-shuhn) Waves of energy.

refugee (REH-fyoo-jee) A migrant person who flees their homeland to escape disaster, persecution, or war.

respiratory (REH-spuh-ruh-tohr-ee) Related to breathing or the parts of the body that help in breathing.

sanitation (sa-nuh-TAY-shuhn) The process of keeping places free from dirt and disease.

technology (tek-NAH-luh-jee) A method that uses science to solve problems and the tools used to solve those problems.

vulnerable (VUHL-nuh-ruh-buhl) Open to attack or harm.

INDEX

PRIMARY SOURCE LIST

Page 7
Bust of Hippocrates of Cos. Marble sculpture. Created circa 460 to 377 BC. Museo Archeologico Nazionale (Archaeological Museum). Naples, Italy.

Page 9
Microscope. Circa 1670. Created by Anton van Leeuwenhoek.

Page 11
Landing at Ellis Island. Photomechanical print. 1902. Library of Congress. Wikimedia Commons.

WEBSITES

Due to the changing nature of Internet links, Rosen Publishing has developed an online list of websites related to the subject of this book. This site is updated regularly. Please use this link to access the list: www.powerkidslinks.com/SOGI/physical